# The Personal Trainers Association
## Professional Group Exercise Dance and Fitness Instructor Certification Workshop Study Guide

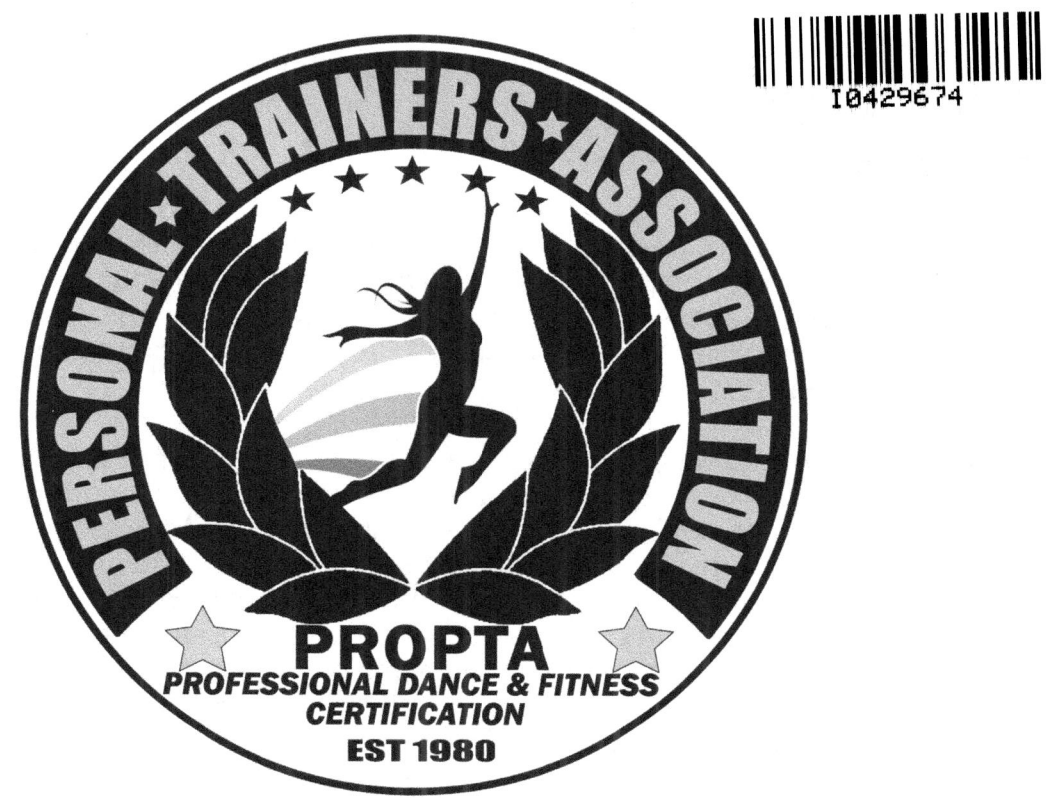

## Author
## Joseph E. Antouri, CEO – CHAIRMAN -- Founder

Congratulations. We are pleased that you have registered for the PROPTA Dance & Fitness Certification. The format and content of PROPTA's training and certification programs are designed to provide an individualized learning experience that will contribute to your success as a Group Exercise Dance and Fitness Instructor. This study guide will be a useful learning and preparation tool when used in conjunction with *PROPTA Scientific Principles and Group Exercise books*

**PROPTA Mission:**

As the world's largest Personal Trainers and Nutrition Certification educator, PROPTA delivers comprehensive cognitive and practical education for fitness professionals, grounded in industry research, using both traditional and innovative modalities. PROPTA upholds Basic Exercise Standards and Guidelines for safe fitness practice.

PROPTA Certification written and practical examinations are accredited by Vital Research and proven experience. PROPTA is proud to announce that it has been granted approval status from the California State Approving Agency for Veteran, and approval from the Bureau Private Post Secondary and Vocational Education approval, GI Bill Approval, and also Officially Endorsed by the International Federation of Fitness and Bodybuilding League the IFBB PRO League, the largest fitness organization in the world that is recognized by the Olympic committee and many foreign Universities in many languages. PROPTA is the official certification of many foreign countries and the Official Certification for the IFBB PRO League, the Official Certification of the MMA and was recently endorsed by the Founder of the UFC Mr. Art Davie.

## WHAT TO BRING TO THE WORKSHOP

- All study materials (for certifications only)
- Registration confirmation
- Confortable clothing, gym attire
- Clipboard or notebook
- Pens, pencils, highlighters, etc.
- Photo ID
- Lunch and snacks (Meals are not provided.)

**CPR certification\*** is required for all PROPTA certifications. If you have a current card at the time of the workshop, bring it with you. If not, send a copy to PROPTA's main office after receiving notice to do so. Test results will be sent via email to all students. Please don't call the office, we will inform you in time.

### Clinical hours:
All students are required to do 20 clinical hours for this course. Clinical hours are hours for practice what you learned in the workshop to improve your teaching skills and to help you pass the practical exam.

Clinical hours must be done with a PROPTA director. Please set up time to properly execute and complete your clinical hours. Call PROPTA office for additional information at 818-766-3317

# RETEST and CHALLENGE SCHEDULE

### Dance and Fitness Certification course

Students may retest or challenge the course with the practical exam only. A fee of $100 US Dollars is to be paid in advance by calling the corporate office at 818-766-3317 to schedule the retest with a PROPTA director only. The written exam can be challenged along with the practical exam and must be proctored. The course fee will never be waived or discounted.

If student do not pass the challenge exams, student must take or retake the course with practical or hire a director to help correct the issue. A fee of $100 US Dollars will be charged for the retake and a fee of $100 US Dollars will be charged for hiring a director.

## ARRIVAL

Please arrive 30 minutes prior to the scheduled workshop time. (If you are retesting, see above.) this will help to avoid delays, and ensure that everyone checks in before the workshop begins and completes all necessary paperwork.

## WHAT TO WEAR

Be prepared for temperature changes throughout the day. Wear exercise attire and proper athletic footwear. Avoid baggy clothing for practical testing.

### Dance and Fitness Certification course

Come prepared for movement. Avoid baggy clothing during practical and the practical  exam.

### All Skills & Choreography Workshops

Come prepared for movement. All students must perform all exercises at all time, no excuses.

### PARKING and DIRECTIONS

It is recommended that you call the host facility in advance to inquire about directions and parking information. Check your emails for such contacts or locations.

### NO REFUNDS

Please refer to PROPTA's policy on cancellation; PROPTA does not refund any money to any one for any course at any time.
### MEALS ARE NOT PROVIDED

Congratulations. We are pleased that you have registered for the Dance and Fitness Certification course. The format and content of PROPTA's training and certification programs are designed to provide an individualized learning experience that will contribute to your success as an instructor.

## Getting Started

1- Before implementing dance fitness into the training program, all trainers must:

- For health safety must answer a health questionnaire
- Must consult with a physician for any potential or present physical problems or injuries and get a doctor's release to start the program.
- A waiver/release form must be completed and signed by the client to waive and responsibility.

- Understand your client's purpose:
  - ➢ *Get In Shape to look and feel good*
  - ➢ *To learn self-defense & confidence*
  - ➢ *Stress relief*

## Certification course Overview

This workshop is designed to:
• Introduce safe and effective Dance and Fitness teaching techniques
• Provide a methodical approach to the practical application of aerobics and fitness theory as it applies.
• Prepare participants for the PROPTA Group Exercise Dance and Fitness Certification exam

This workshop will review:
• safe and effective teaching techniques
• safe and effective proper bio-mechanics
• examination criteria
• practical techniques required for the practical exam
• understanding the body's demand for cardio vascular training
• proper food and nutrition for ongoing benefits of cardio training

The workshop will conclude with written and practical examinations that provide a standardized measure of instructor competency.

The workshop is appropriate for new and experienced instructors. However, an understanding of PROPTA's Basic Exercise Scientific Principles Standards and

Guidelines, successful completion of PROPTA Primary Group Exercise Certification, Practical Skills & Choreography workshop.

The following are a few helpful hints to help you get the most out of your workshop experience. You must not miss any days from the practical application course or you will fall behind.

**To prepare for the workshop:**
1. You have been provide with a *Manual for Instruction,* please call the PROPTA if you don't have one at 1-800-317-3577
2. Read and complete this entire study guide.
3. Complete the study guide to the best of your ability prior to attending the workshop. Make notes of any sections you need help with. There will be time at the workshop to ask questions.

**On the day of the workshop:**
1. Dress appropriately for active participation.
2. Bring the following:
   - Study guide
   - *The Manual for Instructors*
   - Clipboard or notebook (Most facilities do not have tables to write on.)
   - Photo ID
   - Lunch and snacks
   - Sweatshirt or jacket
   - #2 pencil (for the written exam)
   - CPR card (If participants do not have a current CPR certification at the time of examination, mail a copy to PROPTA after receiving instructions to do so from the testing department.) (CPR certifications from online or home-study courses will not be accepted.)
3. Arrive 30 minutes prior to workshop start time.

## Continuing Education Units (CEUs)
CEU validation forms will be awarded to participants who complete the Certification workshop. This course is worth 5 CEUs that may be used to renew other current PROPTA Dance and Fitness certifications previously achieved.

**Step Certification Outline**
1. Registration
2. Welcome and Introduction
3. Explanation of Testing Procedures
4. Muscle and Joint Action Review

5. Biomechanical Studies and Safety Guidelines
6. Warm-Up
7. Use of music

**Break**

8. Orientation to Step-step Movement Skills
9. Creating Movement Patterns
10. Isolation and Flexibility Training

**Lunch Break**

11. Cueing Techniques
12. Warm-Up and Step Movement Patterns
13. Mirror Image Teaching and Reorienting

**Re-test and challenge candidates check in.**

14. Safety and Injury Prevention
15. Study Guide Review - Questions and Answers
16. Break and Assignment of Testing Numbers
17. **Practical Exam**
18. Preparation for Written Exam
19. **Written Exam**

## Step Certification Course Objectives
Participation in the PROPTA Step Certification Program is intended to provide the instructor with the knowledge to develop and instruct participants through a safe and effective step class.

### Introduction to Step Training
• Review the history of the step conditioning tool, and its introduction into the aerobics class.

### Anatomy and Kinesiology Review
• Review major muscles of the body and discuss joint actions as they apply to step training.

### Physiological considerations
• Examine the physiological aspects of step training effectiveness.

• Review energy cost of step training, and compare it to other modes of aerobic exercise.
• Review intensity variables.

**Biomechanical Considerations**

• Examine methods used to assess long- and short-term biomechanical effects of step training.
• Identify biomechanical effects of step training and understand the application of these findings.

**Programming Recommendations**

• Examine program design and progression recommendations for step training.
• Become familiar with training principles that govern program design, including the Principle of Overload, Progressive Overload, and Specificity of Training.

**Class Format**

• Review class format, and identify sequence, duration and tempo recommendations for each segment.

**Warm-Up**

• Learn how to create a warm-up specific to dance and fitness training and discuss safety considerations appropriate for the exercise setting.
• Learn how to incorporate floor mix patterns.

**Aerobic Training**

• Learn how to develop physiologically and biomechanically sound step aerobics training routines and apply principles of training.
• Learn how to create a "bell curve."
• Learn and practice the following choreography development techniques:
   o freestyle teaching
   o block methods
   o add-on technique

• Examine aerobic training recommendations including guidelines for frequency, intensity and duration.
• Review heart rates as a measure of intensity and indicator of fitness.
• Define and understand use of resting, maximal, training and recovery heart rates.
• Understand heart rate reserve and learn how it is used to determine training heart rate range.

**Isolation Training/Muscle Conditioning**

• Examine the potential of the step as a strength training tool in the classroom setting.

## Cool Down/Flexibility
• Identify recommendations for flexibility training.

## Safety and Injury Prevention
• List benefits and guidelines regarding pre-exercise screening.
• Review coronary risk factors
• Recognize clients at risk and provide appropriate recommendations.
• Identify hydration recommendations.

## Cardiovascular Assessment
• Learn procedures and guidelines to implement the 3-Minute Step Test
• Learn how to apply cardiovascular assessment results to the practical environment.

## Abdominal Strength Assessment
• Examine risk and benefit of abdominal strength assessments.

## Flexibility Screening
• Learn methods of flexibility of various muscle groups
• Learn how to identify participants with adequate flexibility of the hip flexors, quadriceps, hamstrings and calf muscles.

## Special Populations
• Review exercise analysis and understand application to special populations.
• Discuss safety considerations and review guidelines regarding pregnancy and step training.

## Body Alignment / Stepping Guidelines
• Define and practice proper alignment and stepping technique.

## Techniques
• Learn room and instructor orientation.
• Identify directional approaches.
• Learn arm movement patterns.

## Teaching Skills
• Learn and practice effective visual and verbal methods of cueing movement patterns.

• Learn and practice mirror image teaching skills.
• Learn and practice methods of reorienting to and from a mirror image instructor position.
• Learn how to effectively preview movement patterns.
• Learn methods to develop and practice smooth transitions.
• Learn to Lead and or assist in any class

### Choreography
• Become familiar with orientation to the dance fitness and training environment.
• Practice the six directional approaches to the step.
• Practice step choreography including floor mix patterns, linear progressions, and combinations.
• Practice step movement patterns that provide creative choreography options.
• Practice arm movement patterns.
• Develop methods of step choreography.

### Music Usage
• Learn the composition of music used for dance and fitness step training.
• Analyze design of music and identify the 8-count and 32-count phrase.
• Learn to correlate music design to choreography development for aerobic.
• Practice choreography development that effectively utilizes the music.

### Instructor Roles and Responsibilities
• Successful teaching
• Leadership skills
• Methods of correction
• Instructor pitfalls

## Certification Examination Criteria

### Objective
1. PROPTA's Certification examination provides a standardized measure of instructor competency. Both theoretical knowledge and practical skills are evaluated in this examination.

2. Examination is based on instruction to average, healthy adults without known physiological or biological conditions that would in any way restrict exercise activities.

### Eligibility

1. PROPTA Primary Certification, basic scientific principles and knowledge of PROPTA's *Basic Exercise Standards and Guidelines* are recommended precursors.
2. Health status of the certification candidates should in no way infringe on their ability to correctly demonstrate required exercises.
3. Candidates who need special consideration due to physical limitations must explain and demonstrate the specific limitation(s) to the PROPTA Director prior to testing.

## Special Accommodations
Candidates with disabilities who need special accommodations should contact PROPTA corporate office at 800-317-3577.

## Written Examination
1. The written examination consists of multiple-choice, true/false and matching-type questions.
2. The successful candidate must correctly answer at least 80% of the questions.
3. The written examination covers material outlined in the curriculum objectives and from the practical application .

## Practical Examination

### Format
The practical component of the PROPTA  Certification Examination is administered in two parts:

Part 1 — Group Demonstration
Part 2 — Individual Demonstration

### Attire
Examinees should wear appropriate footwear, tights, leotards and/or shorts and T-shirts. No sweat pants or other bulky or restrictive clothing may be worn. No hand-held weights or other exercise props may be used.

### Steps
Steps will be provided by the hosting facility if needed.

### Music
Appropriate music will be provided.

## Standard of Correct Performance
All eligible candidates shall be judged on their ability to correctly demonstrate the skills necessary for the safe and effective instruction of training, according to the

description outlined in the PROPTA Certification Study Guide and *Training: A Manual For Instructors,* and as discussed in the PROPTA Certification course Workshop.

## Part 1 – Group Demonstration

This portion of the exam is non-verbal. Candidates shall be evaluated in a group format with music.

### Testing Procedure

The Lead Examiner shall announce the three categories in the order listed below. Candidates shall then simultaneously demonstrate the step training skills appropriate for that category while being evaluated by the examiners for completion of examination criteria and adherence to PROPTA step and basic exercise guidelines. The times listed in parentheses are approximate, and may vary slightly depending on the size of the class.

### Category 1 – Warm-up (5 minutes)

Using the step, demonstrate a warm-up that includes a minimum of three rhythmic limbering exercises, and four preparatory static stretches.

Candidates shall be evaluated on their demonstration of:
• a minimum of three rhythmic limbering exercises.
• a minimum of four preparatory static stretches.
• proper alignment according to PROPTA Basic Exercise Standards and Guidelines and instruction from the PROPTA director.

### Category II – Compulsory Skills Demonstration (5 minutes)

The step patterns listed below will be called out, one at a time by the lead examiner. It is not necessary to memorize this list. The entire group will demonstrate each skill synchronistically until the lead examiner calls for a change to the next step process. Candidates may choose their own arm movement patterns.

| | |
|---|---|
| • Basic Step (Alternating Lead) | • Lift Step (Alternating Lead) |
| • V Step | • Repeaters (Alternating Lead) |
| • Turn Step | • Lift Step-Straddle Down |
| • Over the Top | • Lunges (Alternating Lead) |

Candidates shall be evaluated on demonstration of proper technique and alignment as described in categories IV through VII below.

### Category III – Technical Skills Demonstration (5 minutes)

All candidates will simultaneously demonstrate their own step routines, without using floor mix patterns. The routine will include:
• four or more step patterns.
• an aerobic training bell curve.
• bilateral and unilateral arm movement patterns.
• low-, mid- and upper-range arm movement patterns.
• step patterns from two or more directional approaches

Candidates shall be evaluated on completion of above criteria, and demonstration of proper technique and alignment as described in categories IV through VII below.

## Category IV – Stepping Technique
Candidates shall be evaluated on their demonstration of:
• placement of entire foot on step, without heels hanging off the edge.
• stepping lightly on the step; not stomping.
• stepping down an appropriate distance from the step.
• stepping to the center of the step.
• lowering the heel to the floor when stepping down, except when performing lunges or repeaters.
• correctly executed (unloaded) pivots.
• controlled stepping without bouncing.
• full knee extension (not hyperextension) when stepping up.
• knee flexion that does not exceed 90 degrees when weight bearing.

## Category V – Arm Movement Patterns
Candidates shall be evaluated on their demonstration of:
• coordination of appropriate arm movements for step patterns used.
• appropriate mix of low-, medium- and upper-range movements.
• appropriate mix of short- and long-lever movements.
• smooth transitions.
• appropriate range of motion without joint hyperextension.
• controlled movements without excessive use of momentum.

## Category VI – Posture/Alignment
Candidates shall be evaluated on their demonstration of:
• a neutral support spine — shoulders back, chest up, abdominals contracted.
• a full-body lean when stepping — not bending at the hips or waist.

## Category VII – Safety Guidelines
Candidates shall be evaluated on their demonstration of the following step guidelines for safety.
• Limit single-lead step patterns to one minute.

- Limit propulsion movements to one minute.
- Limit repeaters to five at a time.
- Do not jump or hop down from the step to the floor.
- Do not step down forward off the step.
- Do not "grapevine" over the step.
- Do not step up with your back toward the step, e.g., reverse turn step.
- Do not lower heels to the floor during lunges or repeaters.

## Part 2 – Individual Demonstration (2 minutes)

Each candidate shall be evaluated individually, one at a time, by the PROPTA Director/examiners. Each candidate shall have two minutes to instruct step training to the other candidates, thus creating a mock class setting. A timekeeper will count time starting with the candidate's first movement or announcement.

**Starting Approach:** From the front.

**Instructor Orientation:** Begin facing the "students." Demonstrate mirror-image teaching skills, and at least one reorienting technique.

**Instructions:** Lead a linear progression or step pattern combination with three or more step patterns, appropriate arm movements, verbal and visual cueing, and at least one additional directional approach. Do not use floor mix patterns.

### Category VIII – Instructional Technique and Presentation

During the individual demonstration, each candidate will be evaluated on their demonstration of:
- alignment instruction.
- technique reminders.
- smooth transitions.
- proper terminology.
- re-orienting technique.
- voice projection and enthusiasm.
- visual contact with class.
- attention to technique and proper biomechanics
- prevention of injury

### Category IX – Cueing
Candidates shall be evaluated on their demonstration of:
- clear, precise cues.
- visual and verbal cues.
- correct anticipatory cueing.
- accurate directional cues (right, left, inside, outside, front, back).

## Category X – Musical Adaptation

Candidates shall be evaluated on their demonstration of:
• stepping to the beat of the music.
• choreography that corresponds to the 8-count phrase.

### Score Evaluation

1. Candidates shall be evaluated by a panel of up to three examiners. Each examiner shall evaluate each candidate in every category.

2. Candidates shall receive scores in each category ranging from 1 – 3 as described below:

> 1 - unacceptable
> 2 - unsatisfactory
> 3 - satisfactory

3. In each category, the scores of all examiners are considered. The highest and lowest scores are discarded. The final score is thus established in each category.

The description of the testing and scoring procedure shall not be deemed to be contractual in nature. PROPTA reserves the right to modify the examination process in accordance with its best judgment.

## Examination Results

1. Examination Report
Examination results for both the written and the practical exams shall be e-mailed to each candidate. If a passing score in the practical exam is not achieved, unsatisfactory performance areas shall be noted. No telephone inquiries are accepted. No further explanation of scores will be provided. Please allow one week to receive examination results.

2. Retesting
If you do not pass, you may retest the written, practical or both exams at any scheduled PROPTA Step Certification for a minimal administration fee of $100. Retests must be scheduled in advance through the PROPTA office, and must occur within one month of original testing date. After one month, you must retake both portions of the exam for the challenge fee of 499.00 US Dollars.

3. Certification
Upon successful completion of the written and practical components of the examination, and having provided proof of current CPR certification*, the candidate will receive a wall certificate and wallet card acknowledging his/her attainment of PROPTA Certification. This certification is valid for a period of **two years**, after which time it may be renewed upon showing proof of completion of

at least one PROPTA course or home study, a minimum of 20 approved continuing education units (CEUs), and current CPR certification. A complete description of continuing education requirements for re-certifications will available on the website.

*Note: If participants do not have a current CPR card at the time of examination, mail a copy to PROPTA AFTER RECEIVING INSTRUCTIONS TO DO SO FROM THE TESTING DEPARTMENT. Examination results will be released, but certification will not be effective and a certificate will not be released until a current CPR card has been received. CPR certifications from online or home-study courses will not be accepted.

### Self-Study Outline For Dance and Fitness Certification
The purpose of this study guide is to help you develop and enhance your teaching skills and/or prepare for the certification examination. Use this guide along with *Training.* You can study on your own, or with other instructors. Each chapter (1 – 12) of the manual has a corresponding section in this study guide. Use the fill-in-the-blank questions to gain a comprehensive understanding of the material.

### Anatomy and Kinesiology Review
Anatomy and kinesiology will be addressed: *A Manual For Instructors,* a knowledge of the musculoskeletal system and joint actions is a fundamental component to teaching as it is for any type of fitness instruction.

Review the following muscle and skeletal identification charts and kinesiology questions that was given to you with the PROPTA Personal Trainers Certification. Using your acquired knowledge and/or other resources, complete this section to the best of your ability. There will be time available at the workshop to address questions you may have.

## There are 20 elements of the course that are mandatory for the technique.

1. There must be a proper warm-up.  The stretches will be learned with the movement warm-up.

2. The music must be left on the first 30 minutes of the class.  This is to create the cardio aspect.

3. Abdominals are done at the end of each class for minutes.

4. There is no floor work done in any course. Straight Street is the only class this is allowed in.

5. Routines are pre-choreographed before class. No making it up on the spot.

6. Music is also prepared before class begins.

7. Music is updated every 2 months.

8. New routines are choreographed every 2-3 weeks.

9. Old routines are remembered and brought back to life.

10. Old music is also brought back to life.

11. The clothing should be clean, fashionable, and stylish for your type of course.

12. Women should wear light make-up.

13. Everyone should be clean-shaven, and with deodorant and smelling clean.

14. Attitudes should be positive. (leaving the dirt at home)

15. You should wear a smile and a good attitude to every class.

16. Business should not be discussed at length in a classroom. Conduct yourself accordingly.

17. Body and appearance should radiate health and fitness.

18. It is all about a positive working and training atmosphere

19. The Mic must always be used, with an introduction before class begins.

20. Always say thank you at the end and acknowledge the new students. (welcome them)


## So Let's get started with the first exercise

### Rhythmically speaking?

What is this? Do you have rhythm? Can you hear the beat? Can you count?

Can you clap to the music?

Let's do some clapping exercises:

1. Clap and stomp

2. Clap and 8 count.
3. Clap with choreography.
4. Using the music to count.  The difference between whole and counts
5. The music breakdown when doing choreography. (Knowing your song).
6. Speaking and cueing with music.

**The Warm-Up**

1. Begin with your own personal movement or groove.   The step touches, and grapevines and dances are done before the actual stretching.
*(This gives your body a chance to heat up before trying for range of motion.  The song used for the warm-up should be energetic, and fun. Remember you must motivate and get people wanting to move.)*

These stretches can be done in any order.

1. Head and neck isolations.
2. Torso and hip isolations.
3. Back stretch.
4. Lunges
5. Hamstrings
6. Quadriceps
7. Optional ( calves, or arms)

All theses stretches should be done with music in a rhythmic formula.

Notes:
(Fresh creative warm-up ideas)

# Choreography.

## 1. Traveling movement.
   a. Runs
   b. Chase'
   c. Step Touches
   d. Slides
   e. In the air movements
   f. Twisting
   g. Heels
   h. _____
   i. _____
   j. _____

**2. Making the 8 count.**

**3. Where should it be in the choreography?**
    a. A break
    b. After a difficult 8 count.
    c. Opening
    d. Closing when everyone is brain dead.
    e. When the choreography stays only in one position the entire time.

**4. Combining fun movement.**
    a. Groovy fun movement with traveling moves.
    b. Something freestyled that feels good and looks good on everyone.
    c. Something that you have to use a little personality to look good doing it.
    d. Everyone can do it.

- **Homework – Show a traveling 8 count and combine it with a movement and traveling 8 count.**

Notes:
(Learn to write down in your own language movement ideas)  Show your instructor how you take silent notes on what your minds wants to do.  This is how to remember the movement that you want to keep.

# The Art of Choreography

## 1. Speaking through movement.

    a. Gibberish

    b. No words just movement.

    c. Music stories with music.

## 2. Effort/Shape

    a. Strong

    b. Soft

    c. Sudden

    d. Sustained

## 3. Levels

    a. Low

    b. Middle

    c. High

## 4. Let's be creative with the movement.

    a. Reverse

    b. Introvert

    c. Retrograde

## 5. Where should I look?

    a. The television. Commercials, videos, sitcoms

    b. Children at the park

    c. Senior Citizens

    d. Other classes.

e. Gathering friends for improve sessions

f. Free style dancing at a club

## Dance with Fitness Group Exercise Combination Style

Equations:

$1^{st}$ – The simple traveling or groovy 8-count
$2^{nd}$ – Difficult
$3^{rd}$ – Challenging
$4^{th}$ – Simple traveling/groovy
$5^{th}$ – Challenging
$6^{th}$ – Challenging
$7^{th}$ – Simple
$8^{th}$ – Simple/traveling

$1^{st}$ – Difficult
$2^{nd}$ – Challenging
$3^{rd}$ – Difficult
$4^{th}$ – Simple/Groove
$5^{th}$ – Simple/traveling
$6^{th}$ – Average
$7^{th}$ – Simple
$8^{th}$ –Traveling simple fun.

$1^{st}$ – Simple
$2^{nd}$ – Simple
$3^{rd}$ – Simple
$4^{th}$ – Difficult
$5^{th}$ – Simple/Groove
$6^{th}$ – Average
$7^{th}$ – Average/Fun

- **Homework – Bring a traveling strong sustained routine, No more than 4-8 counts.**

## Do's and Don'ts!

1. Try not to repeat movements in the same routine.
2. Try to have a different story of choreography ideas from your last piece (routine)
3. Do not have movements that look alike in the same routine. Try not to confuse folks.
4. Try to make movement that is anatomically correct. Step right then left etc… No left then left.
5. Try your movement at home at the regular tempo. Try to use choreograph that feels good to the body.
6. Try to find movements that make your students look good. Not just yourself.
7. Recycling choreography is fine, as long as it is forgotten movements from long time ago.

## Arm Choreography

1. How and when to use it?
   a. Teach without the music.
   b. Teach with the music but separate the body parts.
   c. Leg movement separated from arm movement.
   d. Stationary or traveling. What is more difficult?
   e. Not dance choreography verses creative choreography.

## Teaching Techniques:

- Eye contact
- Owning the room
- Securing the students
- Taking charge
- Non-intimidating atmosphere
- Talking before and after classes

- Communicating by using the mic.
- Learning names
- Seeing progress of students
- Keeping your distance
- Energy for the hour
- Attitude: Positive and Natural, not fake.
- Never block a student in the mirror. Be courteous.
- Try to give eye contact on every student. Especially the new ones.

Notes:

## Your Final Presentation!!

- **Create your lesson plan.**
1. How much time do you need to create each section?
2. How much time do you have left over to run the routine?
3. The cool down.
- **The warm-up: 4-5 mins.**
- **The choreography non-stop without a water break 30 mins.**
- **The breakdown and more choreography 15 mins.**
- **Running the routine and no more choreography 5-10 mins.**
- **Abdominals at the end of class 5 mins.**

## *How do I do Abdominals?*

1. Cover all sections of the abdominal cavity.
   a. The upper abs
   b. The lower abs
   c. The oblique

2. The ending burnout the stretch.

## The Assistant

### 1. What do they do?

    a.  They help each student learn the routine.

    b.  They mirror the instructor so that others can see properly.

    c.  They travel around the room to catch all students.

    d.  They instruct the same material when the instructor does not show.

    e.  They are treated like an instructor in the course.

### 2. Can they participate in the class?

    a. Yes, they should be able to lead the warm-up or other sections of the class to practice instructing.

    b. They should assist the instructor in creating    material for the class.

    c. They should always be there to develop a following for themselves.

### 3. The Benefits

    a. They are developing an automatic clientele for their future classes.

    b. They will begin making money when teaching at the beginning.  Will not have to work their way up.

    c. They will get rehearsals before going into the classroom alone.

    d. They get to study under a professional.

### 4. Do's / and Don'ts

    - Never stand in front of a student.  Be courteous.

    - Never give bad energy in the room.

    - Support the instructor at all times.

    - Stand near students who need help.  Not near students that are pros.

    - Give everyone space

    - Care about the students.

# THE SKELETAL SYSTEM OF THE HUMAN BODY

Review the skeletal diagrams, especially the arms and legs.

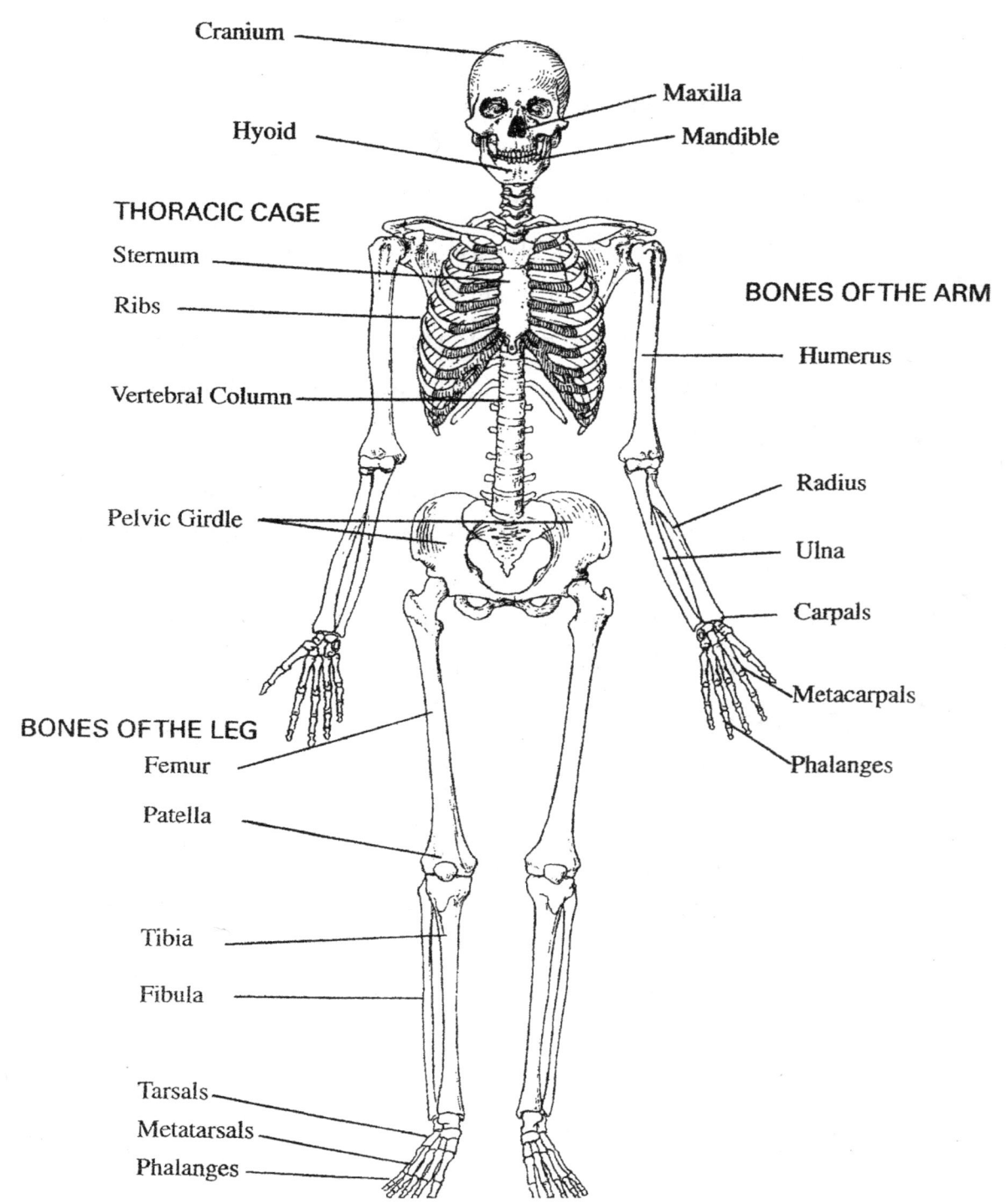

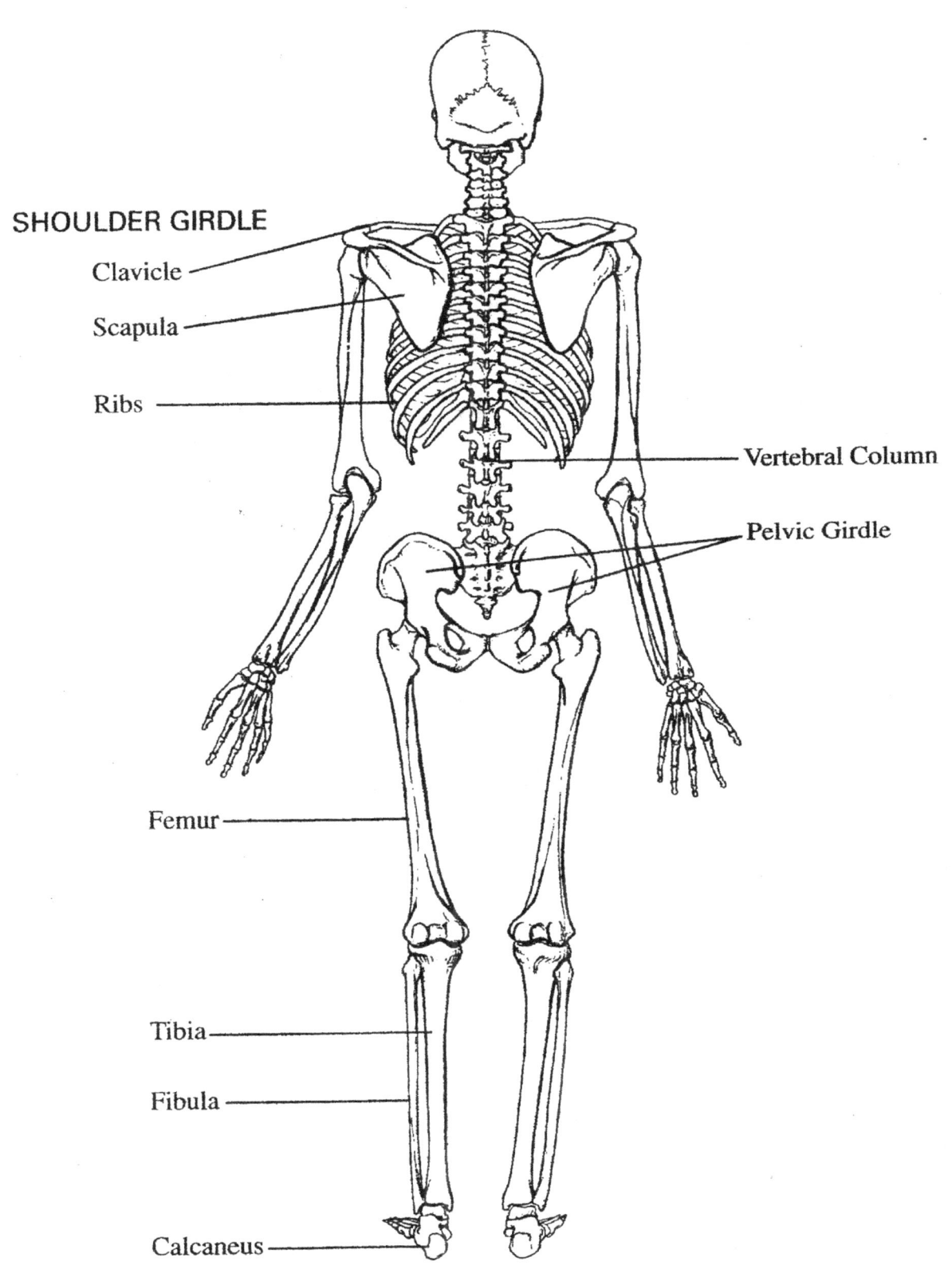

SHOULDER GIRDLE

Clavicle

Scapula

Ribs

Vertebral Column

Pelvic Girdle

Femur

Tibia

Fibula

Calcaneus

# MAJOR MUSCLES OF THE HUMAN BODY

Draw lines to match the muscle names on the left to the muscle diagram on the right.

## ANTERIOR

Pectoralis Major

Deltoid

Biceps

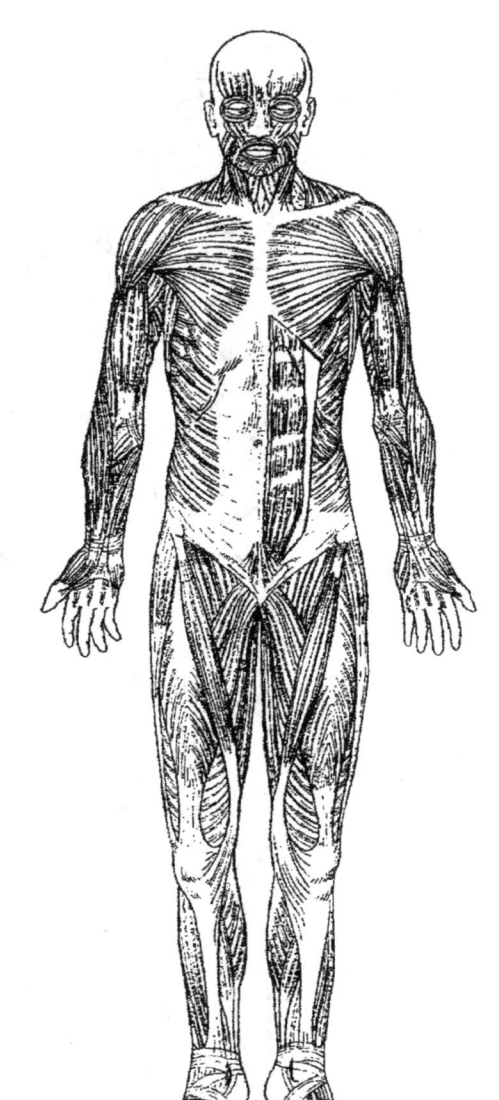

Rectus Abdominus

Internal Obliques

External Obliques

Iliopsoas

Hip Abductor Group

Hip Adductor Group

Quadriceps

Tibialis Anterior

# POSTERIOR

Trapezius

Rhomboids

Deltoids

**Latissimus Dorsi**

Triceps


Erector Spinae


Gluteus Maximus


Hamstring Group


Gastrocnemius

Soleus

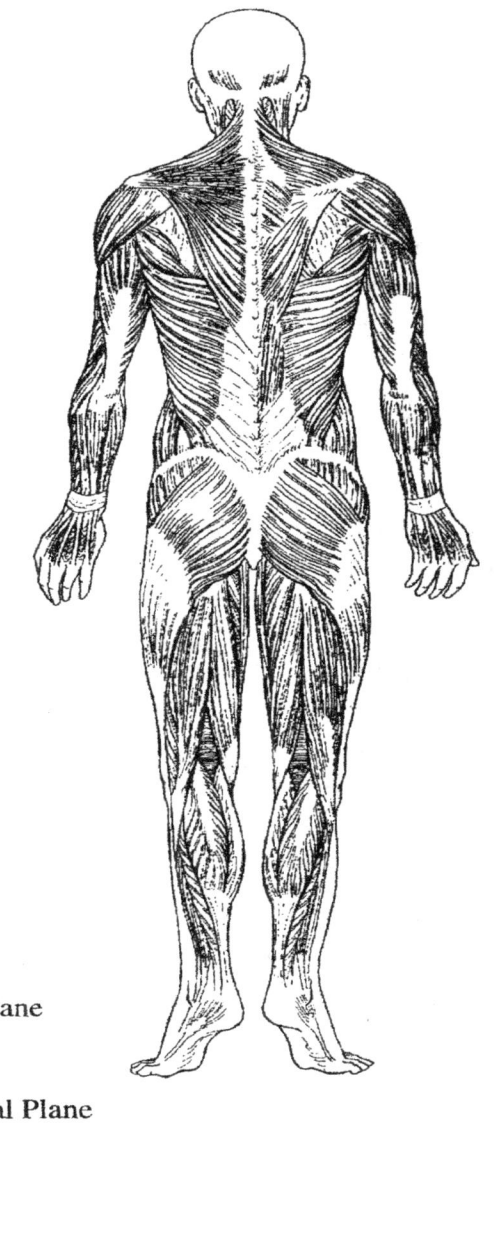

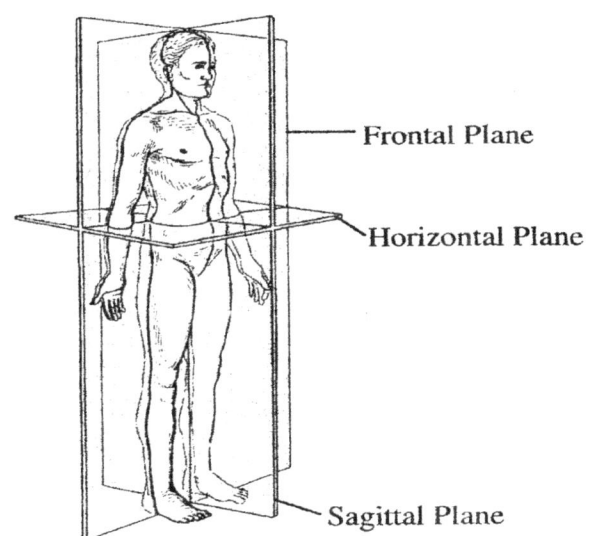

Frontal Plane

Horizontal Plane

Sagittal Plane

## Defined Terms

**Aerobic activities** use the larger muscle groups over an extended time period where the energy is supplied by the oxygen utilizing process. Sample activities include walking, jogging, swimming, and cycling.

**Aerobic capacity** is the highest amount of oxygen consumed during maximal exercise in activities that use the large muscle groups in the legs or arms and legs combined. Aerobic capacity, aerobic power, functional capacity, functional aerobic capacity, maximal functional capacity, cardiorespiratory fitness, cardiovascular fitness, maximal oxygen intake, and maximal oxygen uptake are terms that are often used interchangeably.

**Aerobic conditioning** is regular physical training in aerobic activities over an extended period of time.

**Aerobic fitness** is the capacity to exercise in aerobic activities for a prolonged period where the amount of activity depends on aerobic capacity and cardiorespiratory endurance.

**Agility** is a skill-related component of physical fitness that relates to the ability to rapidly change the position of the entire body in space with speed and accuracy.

**Anaerobic exercise** is intense activity requiring energy production without using oxygen. Anaerobic means in the absence of oxygen.

**Anaerobic threshold** defines the upper limit of exercise intensity that can be sustained aerobically. The anaerobic threshold is attained during more intense exercise where anaerobic metabolism represents a significant proportion of the required energy supply. The onset of blood lactate accumulation (OBLA), aerobic-anaerobic threshold, individual anaerobic threshold, point of metabolic acidosis, and lactate threshold essentially mean the same thing.

**Body composition** is a health-related physical fitness component that relates to the relative amounts of muscle, fat, bone, and other vital parts of the body.

**Cardiorespiratory endurance** is a health-related component of physical fitness that relates to the ability of the circulatory and respiratory systems to supply fuel during sustained physical activity and to eliminate fatigue products after supplying fuel. Cardiorespiratory endurance is often used interchangeably with aerobic or cardiorespiratory fitness.

**Chronic diseases** are illnesses that are prolonged, do not resolve spontaneously, and are rarely cured completely (3).

**Conditioning** is regular exercise conducted over an extended period of time. Conditioning and training are the same.

**Coordination** is a skill-related component of physical fitness that relates to the ability to use the senses, such as sight and hearing, together with body parts in performing motor tasks smoothly and accurately.

**Epidemiology** is a discipline focusing on how diseases originate and spread in populations.

**Exercise** is planned, structured, and repetitive bodily movement done to improve or maintain one or more physical fitness components. Progressive overloading is necessary to improve specific fitness components. Exercise, conditioning, and physical training are terms that are used interchangeably.

**Exercise guidelines** refer to the type and amount of activity specific to the intensity, frequency, and length of workouts needed to produce or maintain desired physical fitness outcomes.

**Exercise intensity**: The intensity for aerobic conditioning should range between 40 to 85 percent of aerobic capacity (1,2). Low- intense exercise is usually less than 50 percent. For some individuals who are less fit, cardiorespiratory endurance can be improved by conditioning at an intensity level that is as low as 40 percent of aerobic capacity (2). From a public health perspective, moderate-intense activities are between 3-6 METs (5). According to the PROPTA, moderately-intense aerobic exercise is between 40 to 60 percent of aerobic capacity (1,2). Moderate aerobic exercise can be comfortably sustained up to 60 minutes if there is a gradual progression and the activity is generally noncompetitive. Subjectively, moderate-intense exercise causes little or no discomfort, little increase in breathing, and should be well within a person's capability.

**Flexibility** is a health-related component of physical fitness that relates to the range of motion available at a joint.

**Health** is a dynamic state ranging from chronic illness or disability to optimum levels of functioning in all aspects of life. Health has been defined as a human condition with physical, social, and psychological dimensions, each characterized on a continuum with positive and negative poles. Within this definition, positive health is associated with life enjoyment and not merely the absence of disease.

Negative health is associated with morbidity and at the extreme, premature death.

**MET:** One MET is the amount of energy expended sitting quietly at rest adjusted to body weight (1 MET = 3.5 ml oxygen consumed/kg of body weight/minute). Also equal to 1 kcal/kg/hour. Physical activity intensity is often expressed in MET units. For example, walking at a 14 minute pace per mile is expressed at an intensity of 6 METs or 6 times the energy sitting quietly at rest.

**Morbidity** is any departure, subjective or objective, from a state of physical or psychological well-being, short of death.

**Muscular endurance** is a health-related fitness component that relates to the amount of external force that a muscle can exert over an extended period of time.

**Muscular strength** is the ability of a muscle to exert force. Strength is a health-related fitness component that is assessed by the maximal amount of resistance or force that can be sustained in a single effort.

**Physical activity** is bodily movement produced by skeletal muscle contraction resulting in a substantial increase in energy expenditure (3,6). Physical activity has both an occupational and leisure basis that includes both active recreation pursuits like golf, tennis, and swimming. It also includes other active pastimes like gardening, cutting wood, and carpentry. Physical activity can provide progressive health benefits and be a catalyst for improving health attitudes, health habits, and lifestyle (7).

Physical fitness relates to a set of attributes that people have or achieve that determine the ability to perform physical activity. Physical fitness is the ability of the body to respond or adapt to the demands and stress of physical effort.

**Physical performance** is the ability to perform a physical task or sport at a desired level. Also called motor fitness or physical fitness. Physical performance depends on both skill and physical fitness. Physical fitness components can include aerobic and anaerobic power, agility, balance, coordination, flexibility, muscular fitness, and timing.

**Power** is a skill-related component of physical fitness that relates to the rate at which one can perform work. Power is the amount of work performed per unit of time.

**Reaction time** is a skill-related physical fitness component that relates to the time elapsed between stimulation and the beginning of reaction to it.

**Skill-related fitness** includes fitness elements such as agility, balance, speed, and coordination. While these elements are important for participation in various performance-related activities, they may have little significance for the day-to-day tasks of most people or their general health.

**Speed** relates to the ability to perform a movement within a short time period.

**Vigorous-intense activity** from a public health perspective, require an energy output in excess of 6 MET units (5). Vigorous nonstop exercise resulting in fatigue within 20 minutes requires a considerable challenge to the cardiorespiratory system.

It isn't necessary to exercise vigorously to achieve better health. However, exercise intensity level can continuously range from moderate and often exceed aerobic capacity for athletes who are competing in sports like rowing, swimming, cycling, running, basketball, soccer and lacrosse. "For these athletes, the optimal range of training intensities should include the range and pattern of intensity demands encountered in competition".

Human Performance/Training-related Terms and Principles

**Adenosine triphosphate** (ATP) is the energy currency for biologic work. The chemical breakdown of ATP to ADP (adenosine di-phosphate) produces an immediate energy source for muscular contraction.

**Mechanical efficiency** is the percent of total chemical energy produced that contributes to the actual work accomplished with the remainder lost as heat. The efficiency for cycling may be 20% while the efficiency for front crawl swimming ranges between 5 and 9.5%.

**Metabolic fitness** is the ability to provide energy (ATP) to the muscles during activity.

**Movement economy** is the energy required (usually measured as oxygen consumed) to maintain a constant movement velocity.

**Oxygen deficit** is the delay in oxygen consumption during exercise when the oxygen needed for energy production remains below the required amount. The deficit is greatest during short-term intense exercise when the energy is supplied anaerobically. This exercise induced oxygen deficit produces an excess post exercise oxygen consumption (EPOC) above the resting level even following mild activity. The EPOC is needed to restore the oxygen deficit and physiologic function to the resting state.

**Phosphocreatine** (PC, PCr) is an energy supplying chemical compound stored in muscle cells that anaerobically produces ATP for muscular contraction.

**Training principles** are guidelines that form the basis for exercise program development. The training principles are defined below.

**Adaptation** is the type of change in physiologic functions that occur with training, rest, and recovery.

**Individualization** means that training gains are based on a person's adaptation rate which is influenced by the type and amount of training stimulus, lifestyle habits like nutrition, genetics, age, sex, and disease conditions.

**Maintenance** refers to effectively sustaining achieved training gains.

**Overload** means that the body adapts to the type and amount of training stimulus imposed and fitness gains are made by progressively increasing (same as progressive overload) the exercise load.

**Progression** is the change in adaptation response.

**Retrogression** or reversibility means that the loss of performance gains (same as detraining) occurs when training stops. Only 1 or 2 weeks of detraining can significantly reduce fitness gains and many training improvements can be totally lost within several months. The fitness gains from many years of training are temporary and reversible even among highly trained athletes.

**Specificity** means that the body adapts to the type and amount (volume and intensity) of exercise load and the primary energy system(s) engaged during the activity. For example, training specifically for muscular strength and power may only produce adaptations to those fitness components without improving cardiorespiratory fitness.

**Perceived Exertion (Borg Scale)**

There are a variety of methods for determining exercise intensity levels. Common methods include the 'talk test', the target heart rate range and the Borg Rating of Perceived Exertion (RPE).

The following article, from the CDC, provides an explanation of the Rating of Perceived Exertion (RPE).

Perceived exertion is how hard you feel your body is working. It is based on the physical sensations a person experiences during physical activity, including increased heart rate, increased respiration or breathing rate, increased sweating, and muscle fatigue. Although this is a subjective measure, a person's exertion rating may provide a fairly good estimate of the actual heart rate during physical activity* (Borg, 1998).

Practitioners generally agree that perceived exertion ratings between 12 to 14 on the Borg Scale suggests that physical activity is being performed at a moderate level of intensity. During activity, use the Borg Scale to assign numbers to how you feel (see instructions below). Self-monitoring how hard your body is working can help you adjust the intensity of the activity by speeding up or slowing down your movements.

Through experience of monitoring how your body feels, it will become easier to know when to adjust your intensity. For example, a walker who wants to engage in moderate-intensity activity would aim for a Borg Scale level of "somewhat hard" (12-14). If he describes his muscle fatigue and breathing as "very light" (9 on the Borg Scale) he would want to increase his intensity. On the other hand, if he felt his exertion was "extremely hard" (19 on the Borg Scale) he would need to slow down his movements to achieve the moderate-intensity range.

*A high correlation exists between a person's perceived exertion rating times 10 and the actual heart rate during physical activity; so a person's exertion rating may provide a fairly good estimate of the actual heart rate during activity (Borg, 1998). For example, if a person's rating of perceived exertion (RPE) is 12, then 12 x 10 = 120; so the heart rate should be approximately 120 beats per minute. Note that this calculation is only an approximation of heart rate, and the actual heart rate can vary quite a bit depending on age and physical condition. The Borg Rating of Perceived Exertion is also the preferred method to assess intensity among those individuals who take medications that affect heart rate or pulse.

**How to Use the Perceived Exertion Scale**

While doing physical activity, we want you to rate your perception of exertion. This feeling should reflect how heavy and strenuous the exercise feels to you, combining all sensations and feelings of physical stress, effort, and fatigue. Do not concern yourself with any one factor such as leg pain or shortness of breath, but try to focus on your total feeling of exertion.

Look at the rating scale below while you are engaging in an activity; it ranges from 6 to 20, where 6 means "no exertion at all" and 20 means "maximal exertion." Choose the number from below that best describes your level of exertion. This will give you a good idea of the intensity level of your activity, and you can use this information to speed up or slow down your movements to reach your desired range.

Try to appraise your feeling of exertion as honestly as possible, without thinking about what the actual physical load is. Your own feeling of effort and exertion is important, not how it compares to other people's. Look at the scales and the expressions and then give a number.

6 No exertion at all
7 Extremely light
8
9 Very light - (easy walking slowly at a comfortable pace)
10
11 Light
12
13 Somewhat hard (It is quite an effort; you feel tired but can continue)
14
15 Hard (heavy)
16
17 Very hard (very strenuous, and you are very fatigued)
18
19 Extremely hard (You can not continue for long at this pace)
20 Maximal exertion

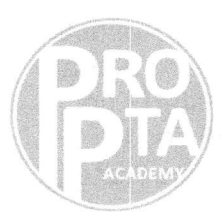 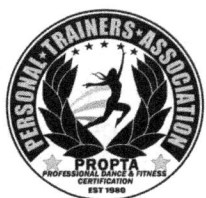

**PROPTA - USPTA**
**The Personal Trainers Association**
 TEL • (818) 766-3317 • (800) 317-3577
Fax • (877) 533-7540
www.propta.com